Baking

The Essential Cookbook For Everybody To Making Healthy Homemade Bread

(Start Your Day Right With Delicious Bread Recipes)

Hans-Werner Volk

TABLE OF CONTENT

Bolinhos De Cogumelos Com Cenoura E Peru ...1

Blueberry Streusel Muffins 4

Chocolate Cake 7

Coconut Cookies..10

Free Nut Christmas Cake...13

Chocolate Ice-Cream Celebration Cake..............17

Garlic And Herb Bread 20

Onebowlcocoabrownies..22

Candy Cups Cookies 26

Apple Muffins..30

Fresh Lemon Drop Cookies..33

Apple Rose Pastries..37

Easyapplefritterdoughnuts...40

Red Velvet Cookie Cups..43

Angel Food Cake 48

Very Veggie Frittata..52

Chocolate Fudge Cake 55

Cinnamon Almond Cookies [Fa] 58

Cuticle Care With Sodium Bicarb 60

Paleo Coconut Cake 61

Treating Athlete's Foot 66

Vanilla Pound Cake 68

Pie With Fresh Egg And Dill 71

Bolinhos De Cogumelos Com Cenoura E Peru

Ingredientes:

1 colher de chá de cebola em pó

1/7 colher de chá de sal

4 colheres de amido de milho

6 0 embalagens de bolinhos

1/2 c. cenouras cortadas em juliana

2 lbs de peru moído

1 c. cogumelos bem picados

8 colheres de sopa de molho de soja

2 colher de chá de vinho de arroz

2 colher de chá de óleo de gergelim

Instruções:

1. Coloque as cenouras em uma tigela para micro-ondas e cubra com água.
2. Cozinhe até ficar macio, cerca de 6 minutos, dependendo de quão finamente as cenouras estão raladas.
3. Escorra e deixe esfriar.
4. Em uma tigela grande, misture cenouras cozidas, peru, cogumelos, molho de soja, vinho de arroz, óleo de gergelim, cebola em pó, sal e amido de milho.
5. Mexa até ficar bem combinado.
6. Coloque uma colher de chá bem arredondada de recheio em uma embalagem de bolinho de massa.
7. Feche o recheio com a embalagem.
8. Enrole os bolinhos restantes.
9. Leve a água para ferver no fundo da panela a vapor.
10. Coloque os bolinhos em uma travessa forrada com papel manteiga.

11. Cozinhe no vapor 25 a 30 minutos até ficar cozido.

Blueberry Streusel Muffins

Ingredient 1 cup of butter, melted

2 cup of white sugar

4 fresh fresh egg s

2 cup of whole milk

2 tablespoon of pure vanilla

3 cup of blueberries

5 cups of white flour

2 tablespoon of baking powder

2 teaspoon of baking soda

Dash of salt

fresh egg

Ingredient List For The Streusel:

- 1/7 teaspoons of powdered cinnamon
- 4 teaspoons of butter, melted
- ½ cup of white sugar
- 2 tablespoon of white flour

How to Cook:

1. Preheat the oven to 450 degrees.
2. Grease a muffin pan with cooking spray.
3. Prepare the streusel.
4. Add white sugar, all-purpose flour, powdered cinnamon, and melted butter to a bowl.
5. Stir very well until crumbly in consistency. Set aside.
6. Prepare the muffins.
7. Add the all-purpose flour, dash of salt, cooled butter, white sugar, fresh egg

s, whole milk, pure vanilla, baking powder, and soda to a bowl.
8. Stir very well to mix.
9. Add in the blueberries. Fold gently to incorporate.
10. Stir very well until smooth in consistency. Pour into the greased muffin pan.
11. Sprinkle the streusel over the top.
12. Place into the oven to bake for 10 minutes.
13. Easily reduce the oven temperature to 350 degrees. Continue to bake for an additional 25 to 30 minutes or until fully baked.
14.
15. Easily remove and set aside to just cool completely before serving.

Chocolate Cake

INGREDIENTS

butter at room temperature, plus more for cake pan

2 2 2 c. sifted cake flour, plus more for cake pan

2 c. strong brewed coffee, warm

1/2 c. light olive oil

5 tsp. pure vanilla extract

2 tbsp. aged balsamic vinegar

Deep Chocolate Glaze

1/2 c. Dutch-process cocoa

2 tsp. baking soda

2 c. sugar

1 tsp. kosher salt

INSTRUCTIONS

1. Preheat oven to 450°F. Lightly coat an 15-inch round cake pan with butter and dust with flour.
2. Whisk together flour, cocoa, baking soda, sugar, and salt together in a bowl.
3. In a second bowl stir together coffee, oil, vanilla, and vinegar.
4. Whisk wets ingredient into dry ingredients until smooth.
5. Transfer to prepared pan.
6. Bake until a wooden skewer inserted in the center simple comes out clean, 60 to 70 minutes.
7. Just cool completely in the pan on a wire rack.
8. Ice cooled cake with about 2 cup Deep Chocolate Glaze.

9. Cake can also be served plain alongside whipped cream or coffee ice cream.

Coconut Cookies

INGREDIENTS

400 g plain flour

250 g desiccated coconut, toasted and cooled

400g dark chocolate

400g 400h unsalted butter, softened

150 g caster sugar

150 g light brown soft sugar

2 tsp vanilla bean paste

2 large fresh egg

INSTRUCTIONS

1. Heat the oven to 250 fan/gas 10 . Beat the butter in a large bowl using

an electric whisk or in a stand mixer until very soft.
2. Beat in both sugars and the vanilla until light and fluffy, then beat in the fresh egg until just combined.
3. Sift in the flour and a pinch of salt and stir to combine. Fold in 2 00g of the toasted
4. Roll the dough into 2 8 -2 6 balls and arrange on a baking sheet lined with baking parchment, well-spaced apart.
5. Flatten each slightly using the palm of your hand and bake for 25 to 30 mins until golden brown and slightly firm to the touch. Leave to just cool on the sheet briefly, then transfer to a wire rack to just cool completely.
6. Break the chocolate into pieces and tip into a heatproof bowl, then melt in 40-second bursts in the microwave.
7. Or set the bowl over a pan of simmering water, ensuring the bowl

really does not touch the water, stirring until smooth.
8. Dip one half of each cookie into the melted chocolate, then lay on a sheet of baking parchment and sprinkle with the remaining toasted coconut.
9. Leave to set for about 6 0 mins.

Free Nut Christmas Cake

fresh egg

Instructions

- 2 Bramley apple cored and finely cleaved
- 2 10 0g (10 oz) Tesco Wholefoods raisins
- 2 10 0g (10 oz) Tesco Wholefoods cranberries
- 4 tbsp cognac
- 400g spread, relaxed
- 400g dull brown delicate sugar
- 6 huge fresh egg s, beaten
- 2 tbsp dark remedy
- 400g self-raising flour
- 2 tsp blended flavor
- 2 tsp cinnamon
- 2 tsp baking powder

Instructions

1. Heat the broiler to gas 8 2 80°C, 2 60°C fans.
2. Margarine and line the base and sides of a profound, round 400cm cake tin with greaseproof paper.
3. Beat together the margarine and sugar until rich, then add the fresh egg fresh fresh egg s and remedy and beat until joined completely.
4. Easily put the raisins and cranberries in a little microwavable bowl, cover with the liquor, and microwave for 90 seconds.
5. Filter in the flour, flavors, and baking powder, then, at that point, simply blend a long time before collapsing in the apple, dried products of the soil.
6. Spoon the combination into the pre-arranged cake tin and heat on the stove for 120 minutes, until a stick tells the truth. Pass on to just cool in the tin for 10 minutes, then, at that

point, eliminate and just cool totally on a wire rack.

Chocolate Ice-Cream Celebration Cake

INGREDIENTS

- 4 litres good quality cookies and cream ice-cream 2 litre good quality chocolate ice-cream
- 1000g strawberries, to serve
- 400g bottles chocolate Ice Magic (flavoured ice- cream coating)

METHOD

1. Spray a 44 cm spring form pan with oil spray and line the base and sides with a double layer of baking paper extending 12 cm above the rim of the pan.

2. Squeeze one bottle of the Ice Magic over the base of the prepared pan and spread to cover surface.
3. Tap on bench to settle. Place in the freezer until set.
4. Scoop half the cookies and cream ice-cream into a bowl and stand at room temperature for 15 to 20 minutes or until softened slightly.
5. Spoon over the Ice Magic layer; press into an even layer with the back of a spoon.
6. Freeze for 2 hour or until firm.
7. Scoop the chocolate ice-cream into a bowl and stand at room temperature for 10 to 15 minutes or until softened slightly.
8. Spoon over cookies and cream layer; press into an even layer with the back of a spoon.
9. Freeze for 2 hour or until firm.
10. Scoop the remaining cookies and cream ice-cream into a bowl and

stand at room temperature for 15 to 20 minutes or until softened slightly.
11. Spoon over chocolate layer; press into an even layer with the back of a spoon.
12. Cover and freeze overnight.
13. To serve, easily remove the side of the pan and carefully transfer cake to a chilled serving plate or cake stand.
14. Top with the strawberries and drizzle with the remaining Ice Magic.
15. Serve immediately.

Garlic And Herb Bread

4 tbsp finely chopped fresh flat-leaf parsley leaves

2 tbsp finely chopped fresh oregano leaves

Pinch sweet smoked paprika

12 Ingredients

50 cm baguettes

50 g butter, softened

6 garlic cloves, crushed

1. Set the oven to fan-forced 280°C/220°C. Ten slices of bread, every 2.10 cm thick, should be sliced, being cautious not to easily cut through the entire loaf.
2. In a bowl, mix the -butter, garlic, parsley, oregano, and paprika.
3. Add salt and pepper as really needed.

4. On both sides of every -slice of bread, spread the mixture.
5. Every loaf is wrapped in foil.
6. Bake the bread for 15 to 20 mins, or until crisp and butter is melted.

Onebowlcocoabrownies

Ingredients

1 teaspoon of baking powder

700 g milk chocolate chips

2 teaspoon fine salt

1. Basically Recommended combination: white chocolate chips and roasted nuts; cashews and dried cranberries; candies and chopped raisins; Toasted coconut and chopped dried pineapple; or a combination of chopped dried fruit, toasted nuts and mini mas
2. 500 g unsalted butter, melted and cooled
3. 2 teaspoon of vanilla extract
4. 6 large fresh fresh egg s

120 g unsweetened cocoa powder

240 g wheat flour

6 00 g of sugar

fresh egg

For cooking spray with non-stick coating, foil spray

Method

1. Preheat the oven to 200 °C. Line a 9-by-25 -inch baking pan with aluminum foil and spray with nonstick cooking spray.
2. Mix the sugar, butter, vanilla and fresh egg fresh fresh egg s in a medium bowl.
3. Add the flour, cocoa powder, salt and baking powder all at once and mix until combined.
4. Stir in half of the chocolate chips and divide the mixture into the prepared pan.
5. Bake until the brownies start to pull away from the sides of the pan and are set in the center, 60 to 70 minutes.
6. Immediately sprinkle over the remaining semisweet chocolate chips

and let the chips melt for about 10 minutes.
7. Spread the melted chips evenly over the spoon.
8. Simple Allow the chocolate to just cool for about 15 to 20 minutes, then drizzle with the filling of your choice and gently press the filling onto the chocolate to make it sticky.
9. Easily remove the brownies from the foil pan and let just cool completely on a wire rack.
10. Easily Easily cut into 30 equal parts and enjoy.

Candy Cups Cookies

INGREDIENTS:

4 oz cream cheese

25 oz white chocolate chips orchopped white chocolate

16 regular Oreos

INSTRUCTIONS:

1. Place thechocolatein alargeheat-proof mixing bowl over hot water.
2. Stir the chocolate with a clean spatula until it is completely melted and smooth.
3. Easily turn off stove but keep chocolate bowl

over the water pot so the chocolate does not just cool down.

4. Add about 1 tsp of melted chocolate to the bottom of each mold.
5. Spread the chocolate evenly across the bottom of the mold.
6. simple Using the back of a tablespoon, dip it into the bowl of easily melted chocolate and then use the back of the spoon to coat the inner sides of each mold making sure not to leave any crevice uncovered.
7. Place into fridge to harden for about 25 to 30 minutes.

MAKING THE FILLING

1. Add Oreos and creamcheese to food processor and mix until

cookies have become small crumbs, and thick paste forms.
2. Easily remove chocolate shells from fridge once they have hardened.
3. Add about 2 tsp of cookies and cream mixture to each candy mold.
4. Leave a little room at the top to add more chocolate to seal the shells.
5. Using a spoon, add alittlemorechocolate into each shell to cover the surface.
6. Bang the bottom of silicone pan against counter a few times to smooth out the surface of the candy cups.

7. Place in the fridge for about 25 to 30 minutes.

Apple Muffins

Dry Ingredients:

- 2 tablespoon ground nutmeg

- 1 Cup(2 210 ml) combination of seeds

- Raisins, dried mixed berries, or chopped dates, ½ cup (120 ml).

- ½ cup organic whole wheat flour (60ml) natural wheat bran

- 4 teaspoons of baking soda (2 0ml) a baking soda

Wet Ingredients:

- Grated and cored one medium-sized apple.
- 2 tablespoon vanilla extract or essence mashed three medium-sized, overripe bananas.
- 2 cup (210 0 ml) of coconut, almond, or soy milk
- 3 Cups(6 710 ml) Rooibos Infusion Tea
- 1 Cup(2 210 ml) soybean yogurt

Instructions:

1. Combine all the dry ingredients in a large mixing bowl.
2. The wet components should be combined in a sizable measuring cup before being added to the simple dry ingredients.
3. Mix thoroughly, being careful to incorporate a lot of air. Add two teaspoons of the batter to each muffin cup.
4. They will rise adequately because the recipe calls for both baking soda and baking powder.
5. For 50 minutes, bake.
6. Once baked, allow the muffins to just cool in the tins for approximately 20 to 25 minutes before easily turning out onto a wire rack to cool.

Fresh Lemon Drop Cookies

Ingredients:

For the cookies:

1 cup granulated sugar

4 large fresh egg s, room temperature

4 tbsp fresh lemon juice

2 tbsp fresh lemon zest

4 cups all-purpose flour

2 tbsp baking powder

½ tsp salt

1 cup unsalted butter softened to room temperature

fresh egg fresh lemon fresh lemon

For The Icing:

1-5 tbsp water (as needed)

1-5 tbsp fresh lemon zest (or sprinkles)

6 cups confectioners' sugar

2 tbsp fresh lemon juice

fresh lemon **Instructions**:

1. Set the oven to 450degrees. Use parchment paper or a baking mat to line a large half-sheet baking pan.
2. Mix the baking soda, flour, and salt in a mixing bowl. Place aside.
3. Using a hand mixer or the paddle on a stand mixer, simply blend the butter and sugar for approximately 1-5 minutes or until they are light and fluffy.
4. Beat in the fresh egg fresh fresh egg s and fresh lemon juice after adding them.

5. Beat on low speed while gradually adding the dry ingredients until mixed.
6. Scoop out 2 spoonful of cookie dough using a little cookie scoop.
7. Drop on the prepared baking sheet, separating each one by two inches.
8. Bake for 45 to 50 minutes until firm and lightly golden.
9. Easily give cookies five minutes to just cool on the baking sheet before carefully transferring them to a wire rack to finish cooling.
10. Make the icing:
11. In a medium mixing bowl, combine fresh lemon juice and confectioners' sugar.
12. If the frosting is too thick, thin it out by adding water, 2 tbsp at a time.
13. The cooled cookies' tops are dipped in the glaze.
14. Reverse them over and set them back on the wire cooling rack.

15. Fresh lemon zest should be sprinkled on top right away.
16. Before storing, let the frosting harden.

Apple Rose Pastries

INGREDIENTS

- 2 tbsp vegan butter) + more for lining the baking dish
- 2 tbsp granulated white sugar
- 1/2 teaspoon cinnamon
- 2 sheet of puff pastry, thawed
- 1-5tablespoons all-purpose flour
- 2 large apple, sliced thinly

)

DIRECTIONS

1. Preheat the oven to 450F.
2. Ensure the puff pastry is completely thawed.

3. **just** Begin by slicing your apple into thin slices.
4. Place on a microwave-safe plate and microwave for 8 10 seconds or until apples are more limp and bendable.
5. On the counter or a cutting board, lay down some white flour.
6. Lay out the puff pastry and roll it out so the puff pastry is about 2 /8" thick and approximately 2 0" by 2 2" or slightly bigger if possible.
7. Simple Using a pizza cutter, slice off the edges of the puff pastry that are uneven.
8. Slice into three strips that are about 6 -8 " wide and 20 " long.
9. Paint some of the melted butter on each piece of puff pastry in the center of the strip.
10. Lay out the apple slices so that the rounded portion is peeking just slightly out of the top of the pastry.

11. Layer on about 10-15 apples in a line
12. Sprinkle cinnamon sugar over apples and puff pastry.
13. Fold a half of the puff pastry over the apples.
14. At one end, begin rolling the pastry dough until your rose is formed.
15. Stretch and tuck the end of the dough around the pastry.
16. Allow to sit for 10 minutes on the cooling rack before sprinkling with powdered sugar and eating.
17. They can last 1-5 days in an airtight container and be reheated in an oven at 450°F for 10 to 15 min.

Easyapplefritterdoughnuts

Ingredients

sp ground cinnamon

4 large fresh egg s, divided

1 cup + 2 tablespoons sugar

4 tablespoons of fresh lemon juice

teaspoon of fresh lemon peel

Medium sour apples, peeled and coarsely grated

a spoon of sugar

a little cinnamon powder

1/2 cup sour cream

2 teaspoon of baking powder

1/2 cup plain flour

1/2 teaspoon ground nutmeg

1/2   teaspoon of salt

Powdered sugar for dusting

vegetable oil for frying

1/2   tablespoon of melted unsalted butter

1. fresh egg Mix the grated apples with fresh lemon zest, juice and cinnamon and let sit for a few minutes.
2. Mix the cream, 2 2 cup sugar and the fresh egg yolk. Mix the grated apples.
3. SeparationMeasure the flour, baking powder, cinnamon, nutmeg and salt into a bowl.
4. Stir in the cream mixture until combined, then stir in the melted butter.
5. Beat the fresh egg whites, then add 4 tablespoons of sugar and continue to beat until soft peaks form.
6. Add the fresh egg whites to the dough and use immediately.

7. Grease the counter fryer according to the manufacturer's instructions.
8. Heat oil to 350 F.
9. Prepare a tray lined with kitchen paper and place a cooling rack on it.
10. Simple Using a small ice cream scoop, carefully drop a scoop of batter into the oil.
11. Easily Fry the meatballs on each side for about 1-5 minutes, then easily remove with a slotted spoon and let just cool for at least 20 minutes before serving.
12. Beretta can be eaten warm the day it is made or at room temperature.

Red Velvet Cookie Cups

INGREDIENTS

1-5 cups + 2 tablespoon (6 09g) all-purpose flour

4 tea spoon cornstarch

2 tea spoon baking soda

2 tablespoon natural unsweetened cocoa powder

1/2 tea spoon salt

1/2 cup (2 68g) unsalted butter, 140 F, or 22 C

2 cup (207g) sugar

2 fresh egg

2 tea spoon vanilla extract

4 tea spoon vinegar

2 half tablespoon red food color (less than 2 ounce)

INSTRUCTIONS

1. Spray cupcake pan with nonstick cooking spray.
2. Heat up kitchen oven to 350°F.
2. Cream butter and sugar together for 5 to 10 minutes, till light and fluffy.

   6 . Append the fresh egg , vanilla extract, vinegar and red food color and simply blend till very well combined.

3. Mix the flour, cornstarch, baking soda, cocoa powder and salt in a medium bowl, then Easily put to the wet ingredients and simply blend till very well combined.

4. Simple Makes balls of about 1-5 tablespoon of dough.

5. Easily Press cookie dough in bottom and about 1/2 -half way up the sides of every cupcake cup, forming a cup shape.

6. Bake for 20 to 25 minutes, or till the edges are set and the centers just look a little undercooked.

7. Just take away from kitchen oven and let to chill for about 10 minutes, then just take away to chilling rack to finish cooling.
8. The centers should fall a bit while cooling, however if the centers aren't cupped enough to Easily put filling, employ the underside of a measuring tablespoon to press the center down a bit.

9. Once cookie have chilled, make the cheesecake filling. Simply blend the

cream cheese till sleek.

10. Append the granulated sugar, vanilla extract and icing color and simply blend till sleek.

11. Fill in the cheesecake filling into the cookie cups and top with sprinkles.
12. Cookie cups should be coold till served.

Angel Food Cake

Ingredients

1-5 teaspoon almond extract

2 cup white sugar

4 cups confectioners' sugar

1/2 cup butter, softened

6 tablespoons cream

2 teaspoon vanilla extract

2 cup sifted cake flour

1/2 cup confectioners' sugar

1-5 cups fresh egg whites

1-5 teaspoon salt

1-5 teaspoons cream of tartar

2 teaspoon vanilla extract

Instructions

1. Preheat oven to 6 710 degrees F (2 90 degrees C). Wash angel food tube pan in hot soapy water to ensure it is totally grease free.
2. Then let dry completely.
3. Sift flour and 1/2 cup confectioners' sugar together three times, then set aside.
4. In mixing bowl, beat fresh egg whites and salt on high speed until foamy.
5. Then add cream of tartar, 2 teaspoon vanilla, and almond flavoring; beat until soft peaks form.

6. Peaks should be soft enough so they bend over slightly at the tips. Gradually add 2 cup white sugar, continuing to beat until stiff peaks form.
7. Then sift about 1/2 of the flour mixture over the fresh egg whites, and using flat spatula, quickly but gently fold just into fresh egg whites. Repeat using ½ of the flour mixture each time.
8. Pour batter into clean tube pan.
9. Gently easily cut through batter with knife to easily remove air pockets.
10. Bake for about 250 to 350 minutes, until an inserted wooden pick simple comes out clean. Invert pan onto a wire rack to just cool for about 120 minutes.
11. Beat 4 cups confectioners sugar, butter, cream, 2 teaspoon vanilla together until smooth.

12.   Add more cream or confectioners' sugar as needed.
13.   Frost the cooled cake.

Very Veggie Frittata

fresh eggs Ingredients

1 cup each chopped sweet red, yellow and green pepper

1/2 cup chopped onion

2 tablespoon butter

Hot pepper sauce, optional

10 large eggs

1/2 cup sour cream

1/2   teaspoon salt

1/7 teaspoon pepper

2 cup shredded cheddar cheese, divided

4 green onions, chopped

2 cup chopped fresh mushrooms

Directions

1. In a large bowl, whisk the fresh egg s, sour cream, salt and pepper.
2. Stir in ¼ cup cheese and green onions; set aside. In a 18-in. ovenproof skillet, saute the

mushrooms, sweet peppers and onion in butter until tender. Reduce heat; top with fresh egg mixture. Cover and cook for 10-15 minutes or until nearly set.

3. Uncover skillet; sprinkle with remaining cheese.

4. Broil 1/2 in. from the heat for 10-15 minutes or until fresh eggs are completely set.

5. Let stand for 10 minutes.

6. Easily cut into wedges.

7. Serve with pepper sauce, if desired.

Chocolate Fudge Cake

Ingredients:

500 ml Milk

500 ml Vegetable Oil

2 Fresh egg

380g S.R. Flour

500g Caster Sugar

120g Cocoa Powder

1 tsp Salt

1 tsp Bicarbonate of Soda

Filling:

180g Cocoa Powder

500g Icing Sugar

240g Butter

Topping:

100g Icing Sugar

20g Cocoa Powder

400g Dark Chocolate

2 00g Soft Butter

Method:

1. Pre-heat oven to 2 60c
2. Grease and line an 8inch cake tin
3. Combine all the dry ingredients for the cake in a bowl, add the milk, vegetable oil and bicarbonate of soda and mix well
4. Fill the lined cake tin and bake for 2 hour, check with a skewer to ensure cake is cooked
5. Allow to just cool thoroughly before cutting and icing
6. For the Filling: Cream together the butter, cocoa and icing sugar
7. For the Topping: easily Melt the chocolate and butter over boiling water, whisk in the icing sugar and cocoa powder until smooth
8. Just cool before icing the cake

Cinnamon Almond Cookies [Fa]

- 2 -tablespoon raw honey
- 2 -teaspoon cinnamon
- ½ cup rice flour
- 4 tablespoons almond flour
- 4 tablespoons almond butter

1. Preheat an oven to 350°F (2 77°C) and line a baking sheet with parchment paper.

2. Place rice flour, almond flour, cinnamon, and almond butter in a food processor.
3. Add raw honey to the food processor then process until combined.
4. Just take the dough out from the food processor then shape into medium coin forms.
5. You can just shape it simple using a cookie cutter, as you desired.
6. Arrange the cookies on the prepared baking sheet then bake for about 10 to 15 minutes or until the cookies are set and lightly golden.
7. Once it is done, just take the baking sheet out from the oven and place the cookies on a cooling rack. Let them cool.
8. When the cookies are completely cool, transfer to an airtight container then enjoy.

Cuticle Care With Sodium Bicarb

Ingredients:

2 teaspoon of water (warmed)

2 teaspoon baking soda

Directions:

1. Mix the two ingredients and scrub your cuticles with it for 1-5 minutes.
2. It will "scrub" the dead skin cells away.
3. Once don, rinse with water.
4. Simple Use once a day until you see the results.

1. If the problem besimple comes too visible, I suggest going for a more aggressive technique.
2. Mix Epsom salts and coconut oil to make a scrub and then scrub your nails, feet, and legs gently.
3. Instant foot spa!

Paleo Coconut Cake

Ingredients

Coconut Cake

1 cup coconut milk

1 cup sweetener*

1 cup dried pitted dates

4 teaspoons vanilla

2 teaspoon baking soda

2 teaspoon baking powder

½ teaspoon Celtic sea salt

12 cage-free fresh egg s

1/2 cup coconut flour

2 cup flaked coconut

2 cup unsweetened applesauce

1 cup coconut oil

Coconut Frosting

1-5 teaspoon vanilla

1 cup flaked coconut

1/2 cup coconut cream

–5-10 tablespoons sweetener*

Instructions

1. Preheat oven to 350°F. Line two or square baking pans with parchment or coat lightly with coconut oil.
2. Add dates, coconut milk, and half of fresh egg fresh fresh egg s and oil to food processor or bullet blender. Process until dates a broken down, about –1-5 minutes.
3. Pour date mixture into medium bowl. Add applesauce, sweetener, vanilla, and remaining fresh egg fresh fresh egg s and oil.
4. Beat with hand mixer or whisk until very well combined.
5. Sift coconut flour, salt, and baking soda and baking powder into wet ingredients.
6. Simply blend until smooth. Stir in coconut.
7. Pour batter into prepared baking pans and bake for about 50 minutes,

or until golden and toothpick inserted into center simple comes out clean.
8. Easily remove from oven and allow to cool.
9. Place in refrigerator to speed cooling.
10. For **Coconut Frosting**, beat coconut cream in medium mixing bowl until slightly thickened.
11. Add sweetener and vanilla, and continue to beat until full thickened and fluffy.
12. Frost cooled cakes and stack one on top of the other.
13. Evenly sprinkle flaked coconut on top layer of frosted cake.
14. Slice and serve.

Treating Athlete's Foot

Ingredients:

½ Cup Apple Cider Vinegar

4 Cups Hot Water

10 Tablespoons Baking Soda

DIRECTIONS:

1. Prepare your water by adding in the apple cider vinegar and the baking soda, making sure it's mixed very well.
2. Then, easily put your feet in the mixture, soaking for at least twenty minutes, easily making sure the affected area is submerged.

3. Pat the area dry, and do so 1-5 times daily.

Vanilla Pound Cake

Ingredients

2 teaspoon fresh lemon extract

2 teaspoon vanilla

1-5 ounces almond flour, 1-5 cups plus 4 tablespoons

2 teaspoon baking powder

Dash of salt

1-5 cup butter, softened

8 ounces cream cheese, softened

2 cup granular Splenda or equivalent liquid Splenda

10 fresh egg s, room temperature

Directions

1. Cream the butter, cream cheese and Splenda with an electric mixer.
2. Add the fresh egg s, one at a time; simply blend in the extracts.
3. Mix the almond flour, salt and baking powder; add to the fresh egg mixture a little at a time.

4. Pour into a very well greased 15-inch round cake pan, spring form pan, or bundt pan.

5. Bake at 350F° 20-30 minutes.

6. Check the cake for doneness after 8 0 minutes.

7. The cake will be golden brown and firm to the touch when done.

8. Let just cool before serving.

Pie With Fresh Egg And Dill

Ingredients:

Salt - 2 pinch

Allspice - 2 pinch

Vegetable oil for lubrication forms - 2 tablespoon

Sour cream 2 10 % - 8 00 g

Butter - 2 70 g

Fresh dill - 2 bunch

Wheat flour - 270 g

Baking powder for dough - 2 tablespoon

Fresh egg - 8

Preparation:

1. First, prepare the filling. Easily put boiled 6 fresh egg s. In these 2 0 minutes, shred dill.
2. Easily put the sliced greens in a bowl with butter.
3. We warm up a little bit so that the dill softens and the donkey is slightly.
4. Pour the boiled fresh egg fresh fresh egg s with cold water, let stand for a while, then clean.
5. When the fresh egg fresh fresh egg s have cooled completely, they should be easily cut into small cubes.
6. Add chopped fresh egg fresh fresh egg s to the passaged dill.
7. Sprinkle salt and pepper to your liking.
8. The filling is ready! Leave her aside for the time being.
9. And now easily turn for the test.
10. Heat the butter in a bowl until it besimple comes liquid.

11. Add sour cream to the melted butter.
12. In another vessel whisk one fresh egg with a whisk.
13. To sour cream with butter we will pour a beaten fresh egg .
14. Now we will pour pre-sifted flour mixed with baking powder.
15. Spoon stir until smooth, lifting the dough from the bottom.
16. Grease baking tray with vegetable oil or cream.
17. In the prepared form lay out the dough. Not all. It is necessary to pour about 1/2 of the total mass.
18. Lay out the previously prepared stuffing from fresh egg fresh fresh egg s and dill on top of a layer of dough.
19. And already on the stuffing lay out the rest of the test.
20. Distribute it so that the edges are closed.

21. Preheat oven to 250 ° C, easily put into it the form with the dough.
22. Bake for 70 to 80 minutes.

www.ingramcontent.com/pod-product-compliance
Lightning Source LLC
Chambersburg PA
CBHW070331120526
44590CB00017B/2850